# LIVING WITH ALS

The Battle of Choosing Hope over Despair, and
Lessons Learned in the Journey

Okey Nwangburuka, MD

**LIVING WITH ALS**
Copyright © 2024 by Okey Nwangburuka, MD

ISBN: 979-8895310885 (sc)
ISBN: 979-8895310892 (e)

All rights reserved. No part of this publication may be reproduced, distributed, or transmitted in any form or by any means, including photocopying, recording, or other electronic or mechanical methods, without the prior written permission of the publisher and/or the author, except in the case of brief quotations embodied in critical reviews and other noncommercial uses permitted by copyright law.

The views expressed in this book are solely those of the author and do not necessarily reflect the views of the publisher, and the publisher hereby disclaims any responsibility for them.

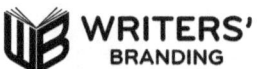

Writers' Branding
(877) 608-6550
www.writersbranding.com
media@writersbranding.com

# Table of Contents

About The Author ................................................................... v
Why The Book? .................................................................... vii
Dedication ........................................................................... viii

### PART ONE

1. In The Beginning .............................................................. 1
2. The Desperate Search ...................................................... 3
3. The Progression ................................................................ 5
4. The Impact on Family and Relationships ......................... 8
5. The Impact on Work and Businesses ............................... 11
6. Re-discover new, hidden or latent gifts
   and talents and skills within you ....................................... 13
7. The simple little things matter a lot ................................. 15
8. Caregiving ...................................................................... 16
9. Maintaining A Positive Perspective Day By Day ............. 18
10. Permit me to share some very personal
    things with you now ........................................................ 20
11. When My Last Moment Comes ..................................... 22

## PART TWO

1. Life as you know it now can change suddenly and without warning! .................................................................26

2. To effectively face new challenges, re-prioritizing, repositioning and recruitment of strongest fighting resources will be required ........................................................27

3. You may be utterly surprised by those who will abandon, forsake and be MIA when you need them the most. .......................................................................28

4. Give yourself permission to cry as you crawl through the valley ........................................................29

5. Travel light! ..................................................................30

6. Re-discover new, hidden or latent gifts and talents and skills within you ...............................................31

7. The simple little things matter a lot. ......................................32

8. Mind renewal and transformation should not stop...........33

9. The disease will affect your voice but not your internal dialogue ......................................................34

10. You need a special someone by you through the journey .................................................................36

11. ALS is not bigger than your life. .........................................37

Epilogue .........................................................................39

# About The Author

At the peak of his career and while enjoying excellent health, this author was diagnosed with ALS. A husband, father, physician and entrepreneur, his life changed drastically as the disease progressed. Originally from Nigeria, he emigrated to the USA in the mid-nineties and now lives in California with his wife and four adorable young children.

# Why The Book?

This is a story of pain, agony and torture suffered by those afflicted with ALS. It is also a story of hope, love and inspiration. There has been a heightened awareness about this illness recently but much is left to be understood about it. There is still no cure for it. While it is a limited recollection of my personal experiences and in no way presumes to represent what every person with the disease goes through, I hope this book adds a little more to the body's knowledge of the disability and loss endured with this progressive and fatal disease.

# Dedication

This book is dedicated to Nenye, Emeka, Eze, and Ogechi.

# PART ONE

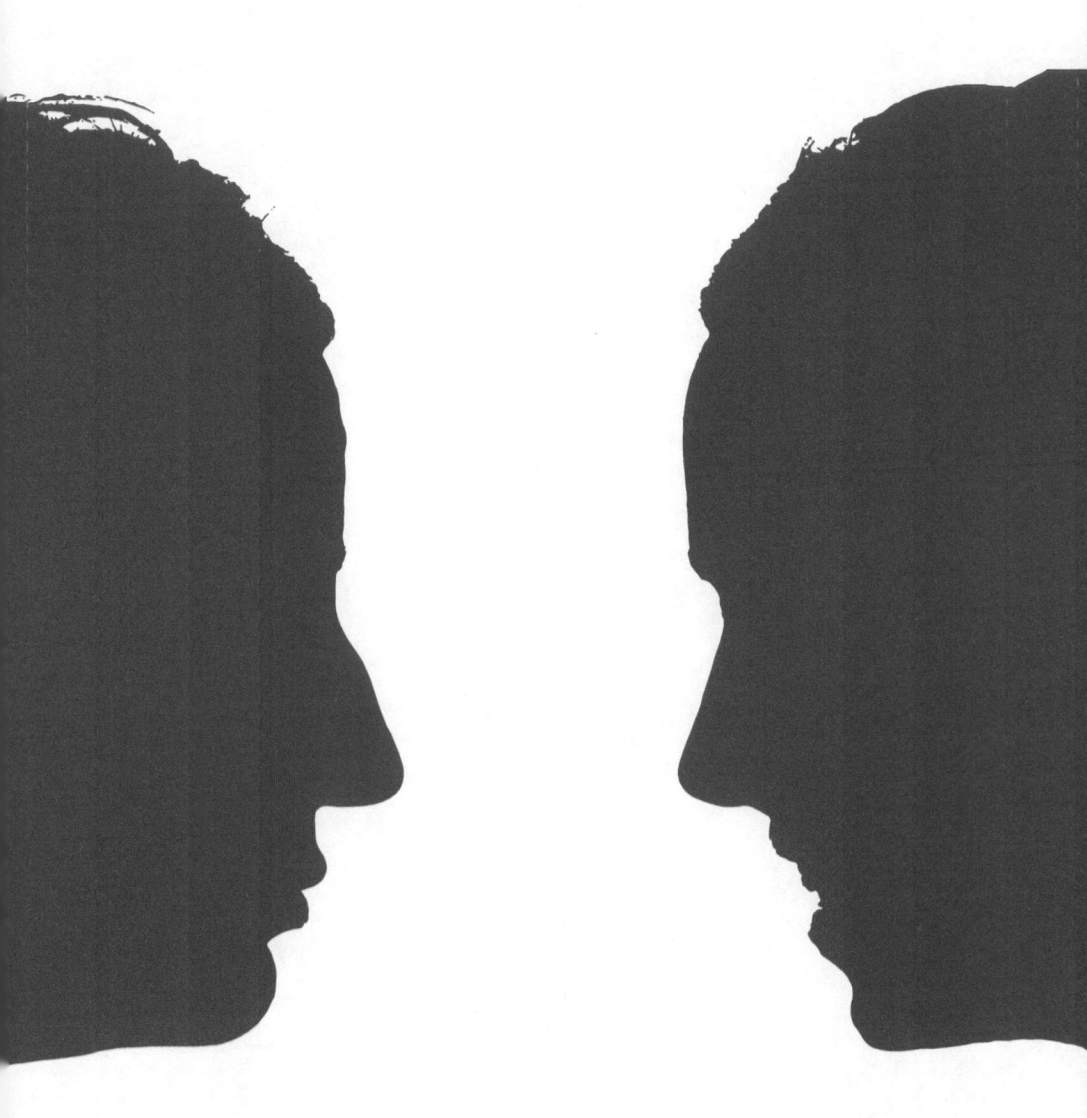

## 1. In The Beginning

By the second half of 2012, I was really pushing it. Working so many hours per day everyday. Serving as Medical Director of a major psychiatric hospital in a large California city, attending to my private practice and overseeing operations at our new health facility three hours away, I was doing an average of 12 to 14 hours per day. Of course, a lot of driving and other stressors were a significant part of my day. Soon, I started experiencing moderate to severe aches all over my body. I took over-the-counter analgesics hoping for relief which was only transient. Adding alcohol to my evening or late night retinue didn't help either. Thankfully my spouse was understanding albeit preoccupied with the care of our very young children.

The aches persisted. Even became more severe especially in major muscle groups. Increase in physical exercise and running miles every morning didn't help. Then, I started experiencing sharp muscle cramps that initially lasted seconds but progressed to lasting minutes. These cramps woke me up several times at night.

By early 2013, I visited my primary care physician. He ran a couple of tests. Prescription of analgesics wasn't helpful. More tests, trials of other medications were not clearing the pain and discomfort. Only a trial of prednisone helped transiently. By spring of 2013, I was unable to make the victory or peace sign with my fingers. I had cut back on long work hours and wasn't driving long distances as much. By late summer, I was noticing mild difficulties unlocking doors with keys and buttoning my clothes. Also, I had difficulty bearing my weight if I tried jumping down from any low heights. Thankfully, my appointment with the neurologist was fast approaching.

That fateful day in September 2013 is unforgettable. I met with a highly experienced and compassionate physician and one of great repute in town. I had gone from the office so I went alone. I was not expecting to be told anything that I would need immediate shoulders for.

After a thorough history taking and physical examination, he ordered a litany of tests including nerve conduction tests, electromyographic study, blood and urine tests. He then called me into his office and asked me to sit in a sombre voice. He broke the news as professionally as anyone could. I could not believe my ears. Up until then I had been in excellent health. It sounded strange to my ears. I had "probable ALS"? I asked him about possible differentials. They were remote, he said. He sounded confident. He then advised I take my family on vacation and do things on my bucket list so to speak. Little did I know how my life was going to change from then on. Little did I know how low my life would be brought in the ensuing months and years.

## 2. The Desperate Search


Before I left his office, we discussed options for treatment. There was only one drug approved for disease at then. After weighing the risks and benefits of that medicine, we decided it was not worthwhile starting it for me. He suggested a medication for muscle spasms. I tried neither. But I knew I needed agents that will help my fight along the way.

I drove towards home in slow motion. I was shocked, in disbelief, emotionally destabilized but determined nevertheless.

I made a stop at my pastor's office. We prayed. I stopped at another pastor friend's place. I got home. My wife and kids and in-laws were in the living room. I went upstairs. My wife was surprised that I came home earlier than usual. I broke the news to her. She was in shock. She cried. I held back tears.

That night, sleep became a stranger. It felt like the awareness of the diagnosis exacerbated the symptoms. My muscles were not just going into frequent painful spasms but now my whole musculature was fasciculating and could not be calmed or consoled. I got off the bed and sat on the floor of the bedroom. So many thoughts flying faster than a ferrari through my mind.

Especially for my kids. They were too young to be fatherless. My wife would be overwhelmed but eventually be okay, I thought.

Despite the fire of fasciculations I felt, my frontal lobes engaged in gear immediately. It was like keeping my house in order while also making plans to fight back with every arsenal that has been tried, being considered for or theoretically make a difference in the prognostic outlook for me.

It was a desperation. One that would eventually propel me to look for and try different medicines from various parts of the world.

Any substance that had been tried in research for ALS, I tried. Any supplement that claimed some benefit for disease, I procured and tried. Stem cell therapies, goldic therapy, stem cell activators, super vitamins, etc; I tried all. Solutions sought from US, Germany, Japan, India, China, Israel.

I also sought unorthodox quasi-spiritual and spiritual healings. Engaged the ministry of many prophets and prayer warriors.

All this was going on while I still worked to provide for my family. All this as symptoms progressed. I still chose to hope against hope and to fight even though symptoms had affected my right hand, right lower extremity, then left leg and was continuing to defy my defiance.

## 3. The Progression

Progression in each sufferer is different, unique to the sufferer. The account herein is a summary of my recollections of how disease progressed from one part of my body to another. It in no way purports to be representative for all ALS patients.

It started in me with muscle aches and pains. Then progressed to severe muscle cramps. The muscle cramps kept me up at nights, would ground me for hours at a time. They didn't seem to have any respect for my doctor's prescriptions until he gave me prednisone which is a steroidmedication. Then, I started experiencing muscular fasciculations all over my body especially at night. It felt like my body was burning up with smoldering flames.

It then affected my right fingers. My handwriting, typing, ability to hold cutlery, and utensils became impaired.

All this occured pre-diagnosis. My ability to lift or have full range of motion was its wicked next target. Following this, I began to lose my ability to bear weight on my right lower extremity requiring me to start using a walker. As a matter of course, I was losing weight rapidly. At some point, I lost up to fifty pounds. Not a huge guy to start with, the difference was very noticeable. Now, I couldn't play with our kids, had to be careful to avoid falls. I also needed help with dressing, feeding, bathing, using the toilet and repositioning in bed.

The progression wasn't exactly symmetrical. By the time my left limb got involved significantly, I could no longer ambulate safely with a walker. I had bought a motorized wheelchair many months earlier in anticipation of this happening.

My tongue began to show more geographical folds somewhere around this point affecting my speech. Likewise, my head and neck muscles. And then, my left upper extremity.

When my vocal chords got affected, I began using a speech generating device. By this time, swallowing had become more difficult even for liquids. I had a feeling tube inserted into my stomach. You can imagine that when my two arms got affected back, I became unable to drive, feed myself, scratch an itch, reposition myself in bed, control my wheelchair, type, or play with my kids. The neck wobbling made it difficult to sit. The weight loss made sitting in wheelchair uncomfortable.

My body temperature regulation became dysregulated. Sometimes, I felt at ease only in very cold temperatures.

I eventually went into hospital when breathing became quite laborious. I got intubated and placed on a ventilator.

Fortunately, cognitive executive functioning and sexual functioning remain unimpairred. Emotional stability is not as unflappable as it was. I tend to cry more easily. But since I lost my voice, I have learnt to make fewer words count when I type on my devive, Since I have been bedridden and unable to dance, I have learnt to gyrate in my heart.

Anxiety comes in waves. Medicines for anxiety have been helpful. As already stated, there is much more tearfulness but no full blown or sustained depression. Energy levels are subpar. I have been gaining back some weight on my new formula.

I am unable to laugh out loud or hard. When my eyes get strained as the eye muscles have become affected, it becomes difficult to focus visually or type on my device which uses i-gaze technology. Lots of Eyedrops help.

Constipation is more of a problem than diarrhea. Suctioning of secretions sometimes can go on for hours. Very miserable feeling.

Now, because of very limited use of wheelchair and being on bed always, it is difficult to go for even doctors appointments talk less of visitations or vacations. Thank goodness, my skin has remained intact through it all.

I am determined, with the support of family, friends, well-wishers to live my best life even while lying on this hospital bed, always on my back looking up. Yes, although it seems I am now at the lowest point a man can get to, toiletting on the same place where I get fed, I am grateful for the gift of life each day. I believe that's all every other person has been given. The difference is in how each of us maximises his or hers.

## 4. The Impact on Family and Relationships.

The challenges posed by ALS could make it become a dream thief, a destiny interferer, business staller and relationships wrecker. Depending on the individual's circumstances, it could also become the catalyst for building stronger bonds, dreaming new dreams, conquering new frontiers and laying foundation for better things that outlast the individual. No disclaimer Xis therefore needed to state that the negative impact of disease on sufferers vary from individual to individual.

The initial diagnosis strikes fear into your soul and could possibly freeze one psychologically. I have shared how I experienced the fears but also the determination to fight for the sake of my kids.

Apart from my nuclear family members and my pastor and parent in-laws, I also shared what I was experiencing with my sisters, a few trusted friends, and some members of my extended family. I found their support invaluable and still do.

I always planned to travel with family as kids got of age. But here I am, unable to do school runs or attend PT meetings at school or watch them at their games. After the diagnosis was broken, I cut back on traveling except if I had to go out of town or country for treatment. Hence, I was able to take our first daughter back and forth to her kindergarten classes and volunteer the mandatory hours at her christian school. The triplets missed out on dad's intimate involvement with their school runs. I do help sometimes with guiding through homework but not often needed now.

Spousal communication and support was great initially but as the practical realities of the evolving needs kept rearing its head, we took a hard hit. Especially after the elder care facility which was established after diagnosis began to consume more and more of her time. I owe a lot for the best she gave. A strong woman. I salute her. I consider this not to be the forum for details of what got us in court and the great distress we had to pass through maritally. I doubt that it would have happened without ALS in the picture.

Family finances I daresay, were affected more negatively by the legal issues more so than the disease and cost of treatments. This is accurate factually until the other competing fact of loss of my income from my private practices is considered.

My cousin became a main rock of support for me. His wife as well. Some friends visited multiple times from Nigeria. My sisters showed so much devotion and love, doing all things asked for and more. My pastor and my local church elders and associates.

My caregivers, office manager and staff. So many prayer warriors never stopped interceding.

Only few friends overcame the anxiety associated with visiting a paralyzed man.

I say that to suggest that the many friends and associates who stopped communicating may have had their reasons but I feel the sense of helplessness did felt during visits may have contributed.

Life goes on. Both for the sufferer and for his or her friends and family. Friends and family will have their own needs to attend to, challenges and life distractions. So they can't always be available. Some may also have genuine and valid disgruntlements against sufferer and choose not to be around you. A respected elder friend whom I had shared so much with told me his decision not to visit was because of those I had chosen to represent me in my affairs. Anothet loved one was documenting my sins for future generations. Yet another went about telling untruths about me for reasons best known to them.

I suppose such misinformation, untruths and outright mischaracterizations arise in the context of an information gap. Thankfully I was learning to forgive all and self though I felt hurt to hear about such from ones I had dined and supped with. It is no longer a surprise that one's worst enemies can be members of his household.

For the remnant that have stuck with me, I remain grateful to, in life and in death. For not considering my shortcomings but loving me even more at a time like this, I am grateful. They know themselves. No neeto mention names lest I forget anyone. To you all I say thank you. And to the others, I ask for forgiveness however I may have offended them. I bear no grudge, malice or unforgiveness towards none by His grace.

## 5. The Impact on Work and Businesses

As disease took its course and I became unable to write well or type, I had to quit my hospital based patient and administrative jobs. I was able, however, to continue my office based private practice because the staff were able to transcribe for me and I signed off electronically. Albeit, my office practice hours were drastically cut back because I didn't have the energy to maintain usual hours. The office work came to an end when my speech became too muffled to understand.

Work means so much more than the income it accrues or the psychological benefits of altruistic giving back, self esteem or self efficacy. Work, volunteered or employed is essential for the well being of our core selves. I believe this applies to wotk before and after retirement.

We were graciously favored as an organization by our major stakeholder who in collaboration with another stakeholder granted us the opportunity to work towards and eventually establishing a sister health facility. Much gratitude to one of the most integrous men alive who has been with the organization from the little beginnings and as Administrator grew the original facility into what it is today. Many thanks to all the employees, past and present, for their contributions. I also cast my crowns to the past and present leadership of the newer facility. The services rendered by them to the surrounding and faraway counties speak for their commitment to compassionate and highest quality care.

An elder care facility was acquired also post diagnosis like the sister facility referred to above. I wonder if there was a sense of urgency in me towards making those pursuits because I had received the diagnosis? Could the myriad of challenges posed by diagnosis have been a motivator in this case?

I had traveled to Nigeria in the last quarter of 2012. I visited with family and friends. I also completed the registration for an American style healthcare facility after preliminary discussion with a friend and brother whose wife was going to be a major shareholder. That dream has been on hold till now because of illness. But I believe it shall be resurrected and eventually will become a multi-disciplinary healthcare facility with satellite operations throughout Nigeria serving both the rich and poor.

I have shared this in part to illustrate the ravaging effect or and the motivating impact the diagnosis of ALS can have.

As I lay on this hospital bed and meditate upon the issues of life and death, I can't help but agree with what a sage said centuries ago that a man would give anything to preserve his life. That true success lies not in the acquisition of things but in fulfilling one's purpose and calling in life as excellently as possible. That serving humanity and being at peace in and out are virtues that eliminate at least to some extent the regrets and despair that contrast Ericksonnian generativity.

## 6. Re-discover new, hidden or latent gifts and talents and skills within you

This lesson speaks for itself.

Times of crises and change present us with the opportunity to rediscover, reinvent and sometimes resurge with new or latent skills, talents and abilities.

Our memories replay our past.

Our imagination preplays our future.

Again, focusing on 'WHAT' theme of questions facilitate renewal.

What childhood dreams did you give up along the way?

What passionate flames of your heart petered out as you pursued other ventures?

What had you always wanted to do but felt you didn't have time?

Your crisis comes with opportunities. You can make the intentional and conscious decision to focus on what is left rather than what has been lost.

This is about transformation.

"My people perish" not because of disease, nor demons nor impoverishment, but because of "lack of knowledge."

God sends us deliverers.

Mental and spiritual transformation requires deep calling unto deep.

We don't want to miss our moment of visitation because of lack of discernment.

Favor is important and can be activated by investing in relationships, making sure our lamps are well oiled, building and increasing our capacity and value to others, by honoring the ones God brings into our lives.

Isn't it strange and glorious how crisis helps transform us?

God trains us to slow us down. He uses challenges!

There are things that look like open doors, let them pass. In this kingdom we don't pay evil for evil. May the free gifts of God not become a source of pride. My intimacy with him is what sets me from the challenges.

## 7. The simple little things matter a lot

Comfortable positioning, adequate suctioning, muscle stretching and massaging, adequate nutrition, cleaning your body aptly, etc and thanking your caregivers for their efforts.

Learn the little things that throw your homeostasis out of sync. Room temperature, bed comfort, positioning and repositioning, how often you get bed baths, pedicure, manicure, feeding times and quantity, etc. Learn to effectively communicate your needs to your caregivers. Help them know how they best work for you.

Maintain contact with your destiny helpers: treatment team, inner circle of loved ones. Typically be mindful of the weak links in the circle. As much as feasible, the circle's primary focus should revolve around your needs, not internal power struggles. Say thank you.

Use the word please.

Do not come across as a slave master.

Also listen to their opinions and perspectives. Ask, tell me more. Ask 'what happens next' when suggestions are rendered. Watch and listen to what uplifts you.

Make out time for meditation, visualization, prayers and positive affirmations.

Discouragement, depression, pain, anguish, perhaps passive death wishes will surely show their ugly heads. It is okay to cry and grief transiently for losses, limitations and uncertainties of tomorrow. Your anchor for these times hold somewhere. Always try to get back to your anchor.

Forgive yourself and others intentionally.

Bear no malice. Harbor no grudge. Love without holding back.

## 8. Caregiving

Most of the news on television, radio, social media and other outlets is mostly negative or sad. You don't hear 'life is good', 'life is beautiful' as much as you hear 'life is unfair.' Is life really unfair? I will leave the more learned ones to slug out the answer to that. But I have to experience that in the so called unfair moments of life, life sends us destiny helpers to lead us to some ease, comfort, hope or even way of escape.

Throughout the course of this journey, I have been blessed with reality caring caregivers. Not perfect. Not always agreeable with me. Sometimes experienced by me in some circumstances as a little insensitive. Nevertheless compassionate, giving their best even when the best may not be good enough for me. I proudly call them my human angels. I owe so much gratitude to them.

My care giving needs have evolved with the disease progression. From needing help buttoning up shirts and pants, bathing, brushing teeth to unlocking doors, maintains ing balance to avoid falls.

Now I require assistance opening my eyes upon awakening, putting eye drops, oral care, haircuts and general grooming, bed baths and body parts repositioning and massage to avoid skin breakdown and to improve circulation.

Tracheal care needs, frequent suctioning, attending to my toiletting needs and cleaning up very well afterwards, feeding and keeping feeding sites clean are also part of their daily routine.

Setting medical appointments, helping me get to appointments, assisting home health staff when they visit, controlling ambient temperature to suit my body, answering phone calls, goint on work related errands, cleaning the house and washing the linens and of course giving me meds. The list goes on and on.

I will not dare to forget the role they play in managing my pain. This they do not just by giving medications but making sure I am comfortably positioned, etc.

Some special souls I refer here to as my psychosocial and spiritual caregivers. They pray in secret. They call with words of encouragement. They organize prayers with prayer warriors. A few visit. Some I call in the middle of the night because I fell or something else and they show up. Some help me with oversight of business affairs. Some advocated for me when I couldn't for myself. And the list goes on!

I owe them all a world of gratitude. And if I have offended any of these helpers, I seek their forgiveness.

ALS might make life seem unfair. These human angels and destiny helpers that have been there for me, whether briefly or sustained, make life worth being thankful. And I am.

## 9. Maintaining A Positive Perspective Day By Day

It now seems like eons ago when the cure for tuberculosis was found. What can we not say about the conquest of most infections. Significant advances have been made in the drug treatment of psychiatric disorders. The diagnosis of cancer does not strike as much fear like it did twenty years ago depending on the type of cancer. Tomorrow, who knows, the solution, cure for ALS may become reality. Those of us diagnosed with this affliction are not unaware of its currently understood prognosis.

Present and constant with us are not just the body damages it inflicts, the Loss of function of speech, mobility and ability to do the simplest things for ourselves. We also live with the fears, the doubts, the what ifs, the why me and other psychological torture and agony that come with it. Yes, we live conscious of the dignity the illness robs us of.

However, some of us know that a few patients with the diagnosis have survived their predicted expiration date. One even became world famous despite it.

So who knows if I may be the next to survive? So we realize you call us dying, but remember each and every one of us has only today and none promised tomorrow.

We are aware that the burden of this illness can be overwhelming but we are still human and deserving of respect. You do get tired while caring for us we understand, but we implore you to care for us and help us with compassion.

Please do not treat us like we are dead while we are still alive, or call us vegetable on vents because you don't know what tomorrow is pregnant with.

Sometimes our pain and discomfort may make us come across as difficult patients, please bear with us and still treat us gently with patience and forgiveness.

Living day by day we are not foreigners to, but realize we need your help. Whatever help you can give to us as individuals or to various organizations that help people with ALS. The ALS Association near you Is a place to start.

Living one day at a time while hoping against hope is energy consuming. But on this journey, unless one gives up and choses despair instead of hope, the following practices I have found to be helpful.

-See it: see the possibility of a a pleasant today and the possibility of tomorrow. See it so much that you become pregnant with it. Remember the story of the tower of Babbel? Even God conceded that if man can imagine it then nothing shall be impossible to him. To the readers of faith, if you believe, the holy book says nothing shall be impossible. The holy book also says with God nothing shall be impossible. So see it.

-Say it; verbalize that which you have become pregnant with. We are told there is power in our words. This is not about denying the fact of the illness but while acknowledging it, also believing for life.

-Wait it out: Patience is sure required in this disease state. Miracles may linger and tarry but who knows a cure may be found or the heavens may smile upon you. There are more than a few that have lived longer than expected with disease. You and I could be among them.

Be Thankful: be grateful for every good gift and blessings along the way.

## 10. Permit me to share some very personal things with you now

They are not intended to be a standard because they are not and oh, how much I am aware I am a work in progress in my Master's hands.

I call these personal mission, vision and value statements as my love goalposts.

Knowing that growth is the only guarantee for a better tomorrow and fulfilling one's goals, I commit myself to some values which I pray for the grace to be God - focused as I go through the rest of my summer, fall and winter years.

The above theory is based upon my presumptions on the seasons of life. First thirty years are likened to spring.

From 31 to 60 years are likened to summer. 61 to 90years being fall and 91 to 120years as the winter and final years of life. Since this is not a chapter on literature review nor of philosophy discourse, I will not go into theoretical characteristics of seasons.

My life vision simply summarized:
- to seek first the kingdom of God and his righteousness.
- to be fully conformed to the image of Christ in all life's domains (spirit, soul, body, wisdom, substance, etc.).

Based on above, my mission statement is:
- to fulfill all my God birthed purposes in Life and destiny!
- to help others find and fulfill their destiny in life.

My Values!
- commitment to excellence!
- Creatively responsible stewardship!
  Compassionate generosity!
  Consistent personal growth and development plan!

Foundation for mission, vision and values!

- Grace, receiving and giving.
- Prayer!
- Stewardship!
- Worship!

Given above, I feel that daily events are under carried by actions and thoughts as described below:

MVP: meditate on word, visualize on word, pray the word.
What things am I grateful for today?
What things do I need to let go of today?
What are my intentions for today?
What will be said at the end of today about how I lived?
I will live a life that when it's over, heaven will rejoice and earth will mourn.

## 11. When My Last Moment Comes

The beautiful journey called life, for us all ends in the transition known as death. Inevitable. Unavoidable. Some see it and expect it to be glorious. Others fear it. A significant number beckon and induce it by the process of suicide, para-suicide or assisted suicide. For some, it comes without warning. For those with diagnoses of rapidly fatal illnesses, their healthcare providers usually warn them to prepare. For those who have gone through much suffering by reason of age and severe degenerative processes, they pray it comes sooner than later.

In severe ALS patients like me it feels like one dies slowly and sometimes painfully each day.

Forgive me as I am not a hospice expert nor am I educated well in end-of- life matters. This is about my personal journey as I live with this disease and the inevitability of my last breath experience.

I vividly recall the moment my neurologist, after numerous tests, sat me down and told me about his diagnostic impression, probable ALS. I thought a demon was speaking through him. But he was a very caring physician. So that was merely my transference psychologically speaking. He asked me to take my young family on vacation, and prepare for death. That night or a few nights after, I wept for my fab four, not for me. They were too young to become fatherless. Hence I decided to fight. Fight for life. Fight this killer disease that would slowly maim me. Fight to live for my kids.

This is not the story of the fight. This is about the impending transition. The medical predictions and my spiritual beliefs are at cross roads. I believe ALS or no ALS, I will live a long fulfilled life. This disease tells me not so. My expectation and imagination is to continue to live my best life while waiting for a miracle cure. ALS says to my ravaged body you must be kidding. So the war goes on. I must confess sometimes I feel going will be better than staying because of the languish I experience sometimes. Then I remember my little ones. And the battle continues.

Healed or not, I am grateful for life. Healed or not, I want to remain thankful for life. When my last moment comes, hopefully there won't be much physical distress. When I take my last breath, I want all or most of my loved ones with me. I want them to sing and cry and smile or lament but in all, be thankful on my behalf. What I say next may sound foolish to people who are not of faith. Faith has been a major part of my existence. My faith teaches me death is transition to a new beginning. I am not a perfect man, just forgiven. I lived to love and to fulfill the mission for being on earth but also made many mistakes. I often missed the mark. So how liberating it feels to have all my shame, guilt, transgressions wiped clean.

Believing and knowing this, I am not afraid. I will be welcomed in death to a glorious pain-free life by my Lord and Savior Jesus Christ.

Culturally, incineration is frowned upon where I am originality from in Nigeria. So my body will be taken back to my hometown and laid to rest beside my father's. My wish is that celebrants, not mourners, wear white and release many doves into the air even as the traditional rites including gun salute for a titled chief being buried are observed.

Am I never fearful of the end? I am sorrowful sometimes because of my children. But he makes all things beautiful in its time. So I know my survivors I leave behind will be okay!

You may be wondering how I reconcile thoughts of death with my expectation for healing? Both contrasts are comfortably in consonance because there is fact and there is truth I believe.

Fact, ALS maims and kills rapidly. Truth, God heals and if we have faith for the impossible, we can receive it. If we can imagine that which seems unthinkable, we can attain it.

So I choose the audacity of hope over the terror of despair! I choose the power of faith over the helplessness of hopelessness. I choose the positive force of love, knowing I am loved unconditionally and all things work together for my good over the mockery of possible disappointment.

When my last moment comes, I want to have fought a good life, to remain grateful for the grace to have hopefully lived my best life before ALS, and after ALS.

# PART TWO

## ELEVEN LIFE LESSONS LEARNT FROM ALS

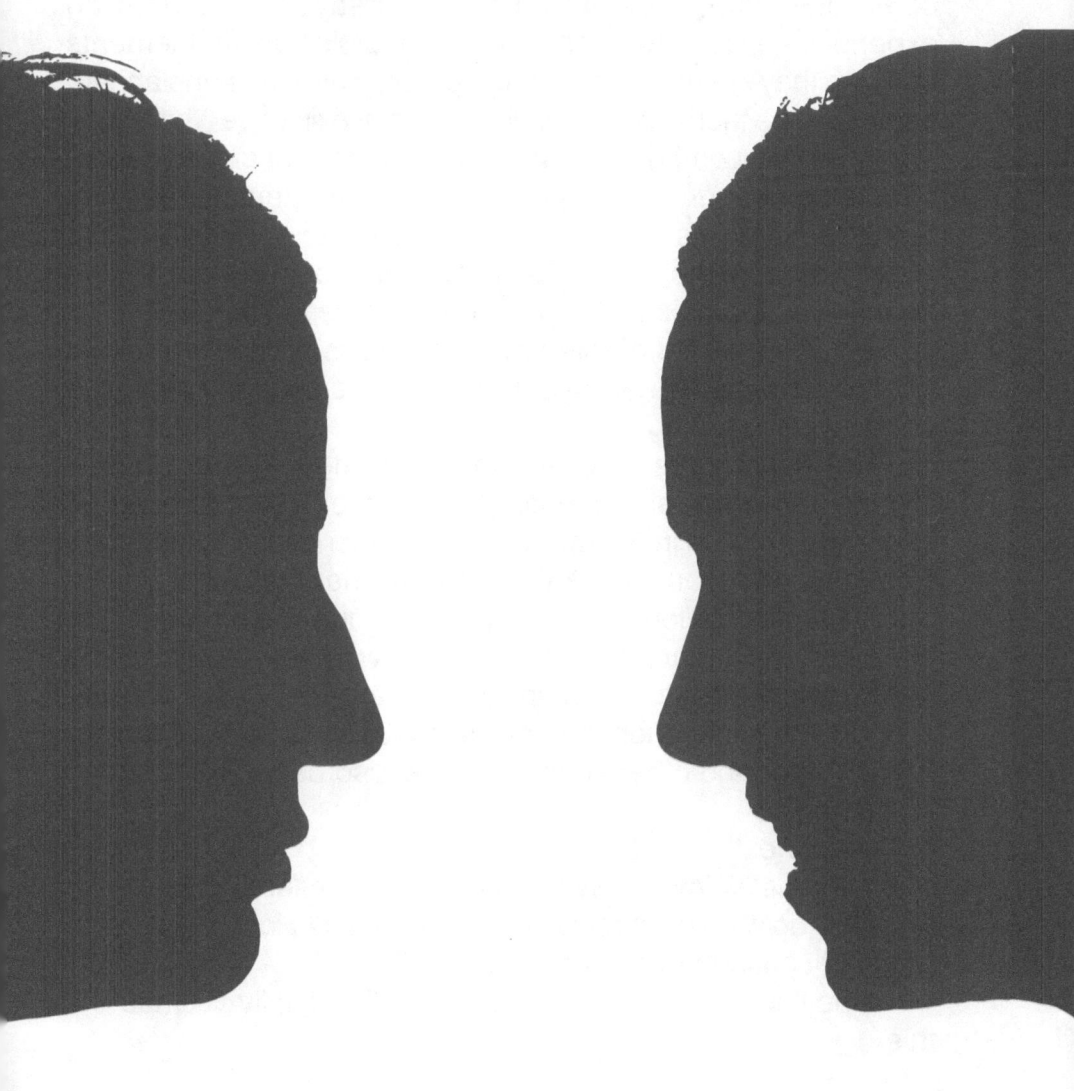

## 1. Life as you know it now can change suddenly and without warning!

This is no mystery. If pre-verbal babies, especially newborns could elucidate, they probably would say: "Wow, what an experience. Due to hormonal and other biological attunements of which they knew nothing about, forces, planned or unplanned, begin to force them into a new dimension of existence where they are mostly welcomed by strange masked faces or gloved hands, people barking orders to one another, instruments of delivery being removed as they make metallic noise sounds and the happy voices of the medical or and nursing team congratulating themselves for making it in a shorter time period this time!

For the parents of this newborn, this is probably a happy change although not always. However, this change came with a forty week warning.

Not exactly the kind of sudden change where a family loses a son who just graduated high school, about to head off to college but dies in a motor vehicle accident. Or a loved infant diagnosed with cancer. A father breadwinner fired from his job. The disruption of long term relationship due to one reason or the other social unrest in communities with high violent crime rates wasting the future of many youngsters. The loss of housing support and subsequent homelessness. The ravages of alcohol use disorder and other substance use disorders. The list goes on and on.

What next?

Why me? Why us? What did we do to deserve this?

How do we pick ourselves up after the hit? How can we start again or continue from where it left us?

One thing is sure: we all need help. Especially at times like this.

## 2. To effectively face new challenges, re-prioritizing, repositioning and recruitment of strongest fighting resources will be required

Crises create change.

Change forces us to make a choice/choices.

That is where re-prioritizing comes in. Re-prioritizing not just our activities but also our values.

In crises, we are forced to re-examine and reassess our lives. If we choose to fight or fight back, repositioning ourselves becomes imperative.

The crisis can sometimes affect your ability to do these things. Recruiting a support group that is able to access and harness appropriate information, offer loving support and presence and help you navigate the best opportunities and path for each involved step is inevitable.

Depending on the nature of your challenge, it may not a fast resolution, so anticipate ups and downs. When my highly respected and knowledge made the diagnosis of the progressively fatal diagnosis and advised I take my family on a vacation, it was like a dream. Didn't return to my clinic that afternoon. Rescheduled rest of patients and drove towards home in a daze. Stopped briefly at my pastors', and prayed with him. I got home much earlier than usual which surprised wife dearest. Called her to our bedroom and shared news. My greatest pain was for my kids, eldest daughter only four, triplets only two.

I was left with only one choice; fight!

I chose hope.

I knew it was going to be a tough and road. Little did I know I underestimated some things that will happen along the journey.

**3. You may be utterly surprised by those who will abandon, forsake and be MIA when you need them the most.**

As my body degerated more and more with time, it seemed like other parts of my life also fell apart. I had destinyhelpers however. Family, faithful friends, ministers and pastors many personally unknown to me and especially my fab four kids provided love, support, encouragement and prayers.

Having tried many medications, supplements, stem cell therapies, goldic therapy etc from different parts of the world, my helpers were always there for me.

Many promises were made by many well wishers in the beginning. Many visited and promised more. But when the music fades and time lapses and dusk draws near, only a faithful few will remain.

Do not be surprised, shocked, discouraged or dismayed to find out that some you believed will always stand by you will be missing in action.

Do not be downcast to learn that some you trusted, ate, drank and played with will spread unfounded lies against you. Sometimes as they say, such is life.

Do not focus your energy on the disappointments that may come from members of your innermost circle or your household. You cannot afford the distraction. Your energy should be directed towards love, forgiveness, seeking mercy and repentance.

The handful of faithful few will be enough even when it does not seem like it. Remember some are in your life for a season. Only God can meet all your needs. No man or woman can.

## 4. Give yourself permission to cry as you crawl through the valley

To receive relevant help and to come to terms with your new limitations. But do not let your self become lost or make demigods of your helpers.

How easy it is for well meaning friends to ask you to be strong and not cry in your situation. They mean well. Sometimes their advice is borne out of the anxiety provoked within them that they are not able to manage.

Cry if you must!

Beat up a pillow!

Take martial arts classes if it suits you!

Running, pottery, biking, golf, etc. Whatever sublimates that raw energy into a more concretized circumscribed form.

But don't stop there.

Reassess what you have left, not what has been taken by the challenge.

Our new victory comes from what is left : physically, intellectually, spiritually, emotionally, financially, domestically and materially.

What do you have left? Take a written inventory.

Wait, weigh options, give thanks and start afresh.

## 5. Travel light!

Forgive and ask for forgiveness. Offload all unnecessary baggage from the past, through your anguish draw from whatever well of joy in you today, tomorrow when it comes is a precious gift to be thankful for.

This lesson speaks easy but can be tenuos. It calls for our openness to be broken and our pride crushed.

You may genuinely feel a right to avenge, curse the day you were born, lash out at backstabbing unfriendly friends or even at God.

Broken dreams, shattered dreams, feelings of rage, helplessness and hopelessness bring you to the place of asking existential questions.

Why am I here?

Where from came or evolved I?

Any purpose or meaning to this?

How you navigate these questions now or did before the onslaught of crisis can influence the pathway for your journey forward.

Brokenness, contriteness, laying aside narcissistic egocentric self for a different experience of healthier humble and grateful self that recognizes that you are not all that and some more if not for the sacrificial help of many before you is not an easy pill to swallow. But choosing this travel path brings peace and uncommon comfort.

No wonder the common saying, "crises can make us bitter or better!"

The journey maybe longer than expected: travel as light as you can. Take the fruits borne out of your brokenness, will be useful tools for helping others along the way.

## 6. Re-discover new, hidden or latent gifts and talents and skills within you

This lesson speaks for itself. Times of crises and change present us with the opportunity to rediscover, reinvent and sometimes resurge with new or latent skills, talents and abilities.

Our memories replay our past.

Our imagination preplays our future.

Again, focusing on 'WHAT' theme of questions facilitate renewal.

What childhood dreams did you give up along the way?

What passionate flames of your heart petered out as you pursued other ventures?

What had you always wanted to do but felt you didn't have time?

Your crisis comes with opportunities. You can make the intentional and conscious decision to focus on what is left rather than what has been lost.

## 7. The simple little things matter a lot.

Comfortable positioning, adequate suctioning, muscle stretching and massaging, adequate nutrition, cleaning your body aptly, etc and thanking your caregivers for their efforts.

Learn the little things that throw your homeostasis out of sync. Room temperature, bed comfort, positioning and repositioning, how often you get bed baths, pedicure, manicure, feeding times and quantity, etc. Learn to effectively communicate your needs to your caregivers. Help them know how they best work for you.

Maintain contact with your destiny helpers: treatment team and inner circle of loved ones. Typically, be mindful of the weak links in the circle. As much as feasible, the circle's primary focus should revolve around your needs, not internal power struggles. Say thank you.

Use the word please.

Do not come across as a slave master.

Also listen to their opinions and perspectives. Ask, tell me more. Ask 'what happens next' when suggestions are rendered. Watch and listen to what uplifts you.

Make out time for meditation, visualization, prayers and positive affirmations.

Discouragement, depression, pain, anguish, perhaps passive death wishes will surely show their ugly heads. Ok to cry and grief transiently for losses, limitations and uncertainties of tomorrow. Your anchor for these times hold somewhere. Always try to get back to your anchor.

Forgive yourself and others intentionally.

Bear no malice. Harbor no grudge. Love without holding back.

## 8. Mind renewal and transformation should not stop

The more you body is broken down by disease, let your spirit soar on positive promises.

Time was when tuberculosis was a death sentence.

Not long ago, AIDS/HIV was also a death sentence.

Today, many forms of cancer are treatable.

Today, ALS is considered progressively fatal. The few approved medications offer less than minimal hope for a few more months of life at best.

But tomorrow is certainly pregnant with possibilities.

Besides, despite the poor prognosis a few people mostly unknown have survived disease for decades. In no way am I attempting to inspire false hope among ALS patients, but truth is, there is a small percentage of people who survive longer than the average doctor's prognostic guess of time of expiration.

Family loving support, patients' will to live have been attributed to this observation of resilience.

What does above have to do with mind transformation?

As a man thinketh in his heart so is he.

Opening up oneself to the possibility of the impossible while ready for the prognosticated worst is a viable option.

To fight in wisdom rather than throwing in the towel.

Our bodies have self reparative and healing properties, certainly not well studied in ALS but applicable to all human conditions. Opening up our minds to the possibility of "a miracle" can be helpful. Awakening our spiritual and untapped mental resourcesto the unusual and unexpected. Utilizing complementary and alternative unorthodox but unharmful treatments may increase your fighting chance.

At the end you want to be able to say "I fought a good fight" for the sake of my loved ones.

## 9. The disease will affect your voice but not your internal dialogue

Focus on your belief, not only what the doctors say.

Your challenges, crises or changes may reduce you to a state of voiceless helplessness. You could be brought so low that you practically depend on others for virtually everything.

Whatever we focus on enlarges. I know it is impossible to be unaware of the pain, anguish, limitations and impairments that have resulted from the crisis. Some challenges may impact your biological ability to self regulate appropriately. When that is not the case, consciously trying to deconstruct and reframe the WHY questions to WHAT questions become very essential. Likewise changing your internal dialogue continually. As well as maintaining a positive attitude of expectancy regarding our desires even if those desires are contrary to the doctor's prognosis.

How you think about stress is as important if not more important than the biological impact of the stress. See the stress associated with your challenges as an ally.

Your nervous system responds to the words of your inner voice. Think and speak to and visualize your desire (healing, change, stability and newness).

Do not dwell on the seemingly impossible or negative symptoms.

When thoughts, images and anxieties about your condition seem to want to overwhelm you, flash out your positive affirmations and verbalize them, repeat over and over until your consciousness and subconsciousness are almost on same page regarding affirmation.

Ask WHAT questions rather than WHY ME questions. What strengths, virtues and vision remain despite crisis. How can what is left be maximized fully? Maybe to compensate for those currently lost or unacceptable?

Remember to recruit the help of those who believe in your goals to assist. Not everyone around you believes like you do.

Stay single eyed. Stay focused on the results you are believing for. Life gives us what we believe, not what we 'want'!

## 10. You need a special someone by you through the journey

Yes, there will be destiny helpers but a loving caring lover makes journey easier.

Quality vertical and horizontal relationships are the sole and soul of happiness in life!

But quality romantic relationship is the cement that binds the involved hearts going through the loss or pain or challenge that enables them create new memories, imagine success, support each other and inspire to keep pushing.

Caregivers can go above and beyond, care for you with all they have and how enriching and refreshing that can be. But it never equals that touch, that look in the eyes of a romantically loved mate.

Romance in this instance is not over rated. One could have genuinely caring friends with benefits but they won't be able to fill the void if true romantic love does not exist. Is it possibly why the covenant of love between partners buffers and cushions them through most stressors?

My marriage was under extreme pressure during this sojourn. Who knows what impact could have otherwise been made. I was also praying for the impossible so I kept potential romantic pursuits at bay.

Pain, change, challenge, issues and difficulties are better endured if a patient, long suffering romantic partner is there to bring solace, comfort and even gentle rebuke sometimes.

A quality relationship, romantic or not, will add value to your life, involve sacrifice, energy and time investments from the partners.

Beware of those who profess their love and devotion in your presence but behind they devalue and dishonor you.

Remember, on the best days of your partner, they cannot meet all your needs. Only God can.

## 11. ALS is not bigger than your life.

Everyone born on earth is dying. When your time comes to go, as much as possible, look back and give thanks for every meaningful relationship and for fighting a good fight!
I have fought a good fight.
Rather should have said I am fighting a good fight.
Better still, I am being helped to fight a good fight.
I have always had help although not always conscious of it. Before the challenges, during the challenges and after it is all over, I know from my innermost wells and bowels that I will give thanks for all the help divinely sent my way.
The day or the hour I don't know. The period or time frame for my transition my inner being will receive illumination. I am therefore neither anxious or afraid. Transitions usually imply elevation. I believe in a material after life in the spiritual planes. Sounds oxymoronic to some? It's not. It doesn't matter anyway. Matter does not simply cease to exist. I am at peace. Peace on the inside. Peace outwardly. When the moment to finally close my eyes to this dimension and open them to another, I pray to be with my loved ones.
For through a challenge or not, it will come.
The Spirit of spirits bears witness with my spirit that I will be helped into All Light by His everlasting arms.
Naked I came.
Naked will I return.
Bank accounts, zip codes of residence, cars and other possessions won't count. Lives positively impacted for the kingdom will be all that is relevant.
So, loved ones, cry if you must. But celebrate that grace that was more than sufficient for me. The Love that umbrella'd me daily. The Mercy that followed me everyday. The Blood that spoke better things and canceled all ordinances written against me. The Word of my mouth that agreed with His Word and

overcame the enemy. The Spirit that moved upon the surface of my challenges and turned darkness into light.

Yes, celebrate. Mourn. But life goes on. Who knows who will come next.

When your time comes, may it be in ripe full age. May you have stored treasures above. May your stars be many.

## Epilogue

Resources

-Your primary health care provider (MD, DO, NP/PA)
-Your general neurologist
-Your ALS neurologist
-ALS associations
-Family, friends, well wishers and local faith community
-ALSTDI
-www.clinicaltrials.gov

## END

www.ingramcontent.com/pod-product-compliance
Lightning Source LLC
LaVergne TN
LVHW041558070526
838199LV00046B/2035